The Purpose of this Book

Every year tens of thousands of people including doctors, medical students, paramedics, nurses, nursing students, and others involved in the care and treatment of cardiac patients, get introduced to echocardiography; aka Echo or Ultrasound of the Heart.

The principles of echo are founded in physics although the interpretation of the results, e.g. color flow echo, shows that the use of Doppler shift and the direction of blood flow was not fully appreciated by those developing Cardiac Echo. Nonetheless, the principles remain the same and this book will provide you with the basic information you need to know, to understand Cardiac Echo.

This book in the series on Echocardiograms is designed for Nurses, Nursing Students and Nurse Practitioners.

Interpreting Echocardiograms for Nurses, Nursing Students & Nurse Practitioners.

By: Dr. Richard M. Fleming
Physicist – Nuclear Cardiologist

Sometimes Learning is Painful Because we are Distracted or not Listening.

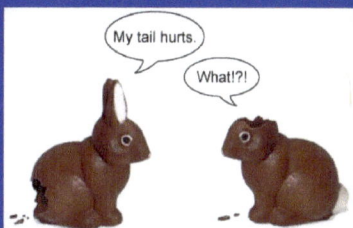

Echocardiograms are Diagnostic, Not Therapeutic!

- Ordering studies are for diagnostic purposes.
  - They are not therapeutic.
  - They should only be ordered to answer questions you don't have answers to, not just to get a number.
    - Patients in heart failure are in heart failure. Knowing the exact % EF doesn't (or at least shouldn't) change your treatment of someone.
    - You hear a murmur. You shouldn't need an echocardiogram to tell you what the murmur is.
    - Echocardiograms do NOT rule out endocarditis.

Position of the Heart in Your Chest.

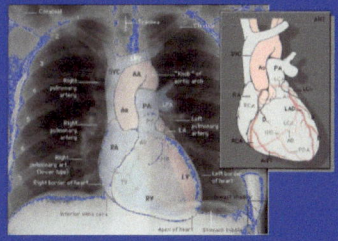 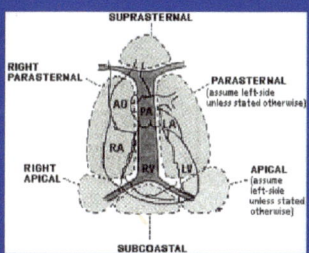

What is Echocardiography?

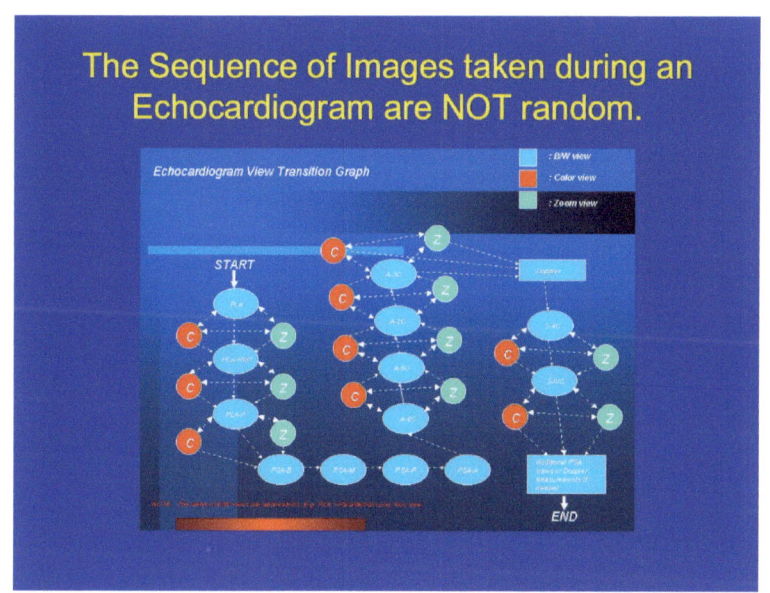

Where you look on an Echocardiogram determines what you can see.

- Parasternal
  - Long axis
  - Short axis
- Apical
  - Four chamber
  - Five chamber
  - Two chamber
- Sub-xiphoid
- Suprasternal notch

- Chamber sizes
- Appearance of the valves
  - Thickening
  - Regurgitation
  - Stenosis
- Wall motion
  - Systolic
  - Diastolic
- Pressures

Parasternal Long Axis View

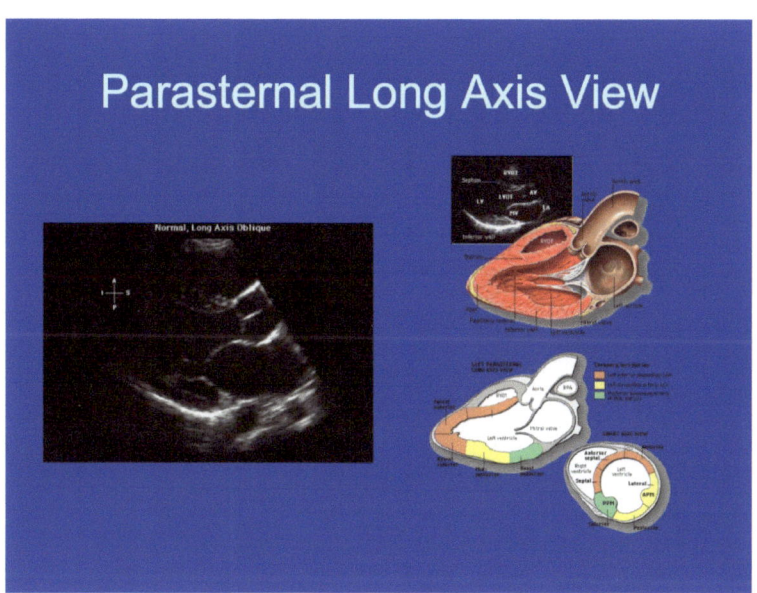

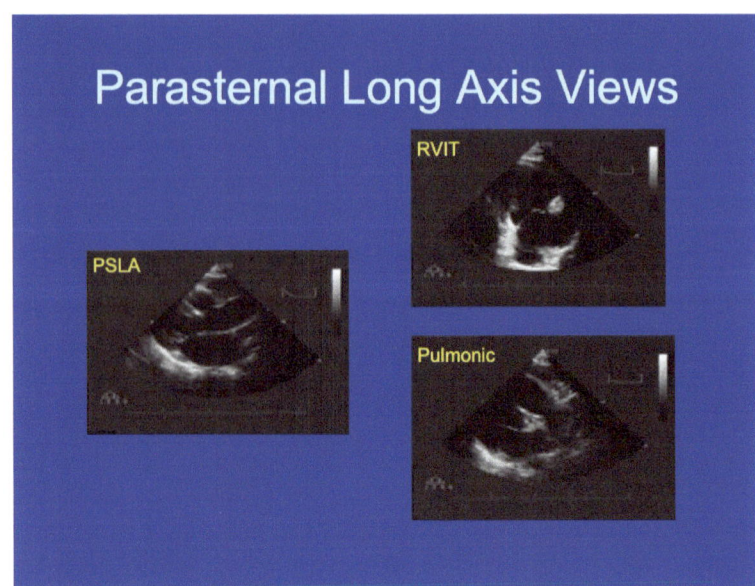

Parasternal Short-Axis

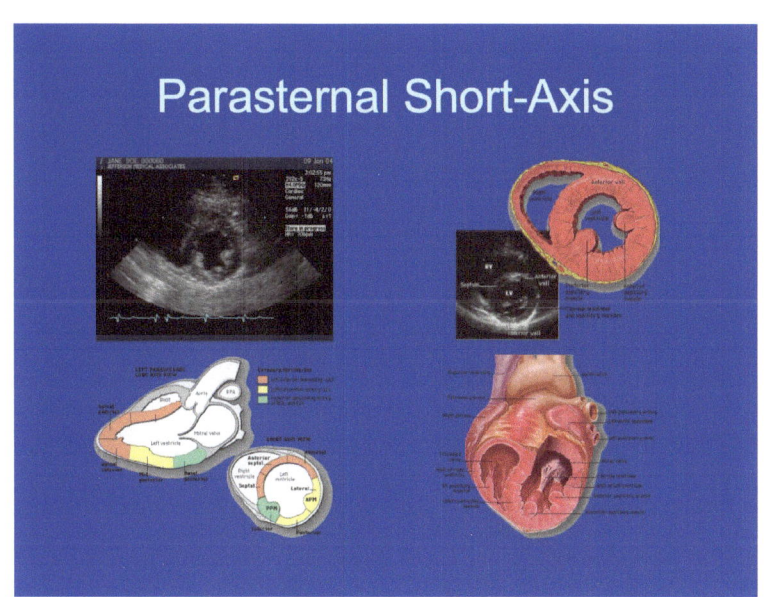

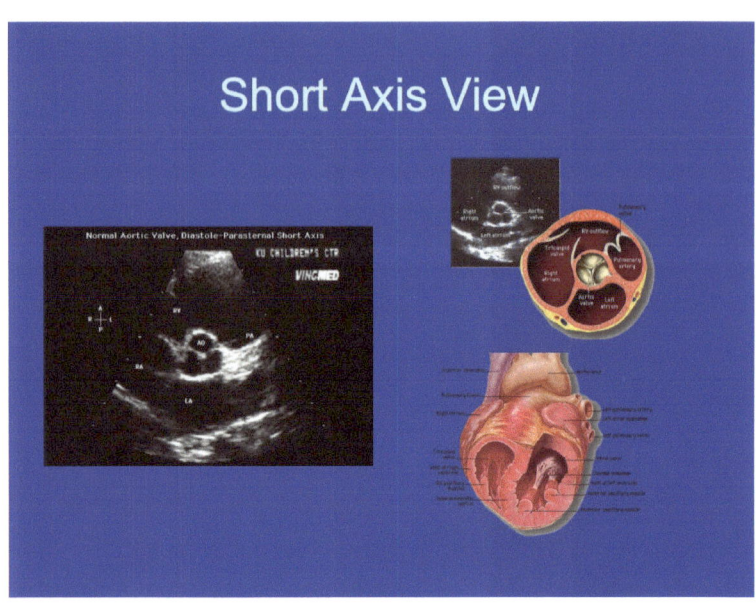

Parasternal Short Axis Views

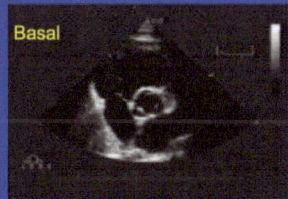 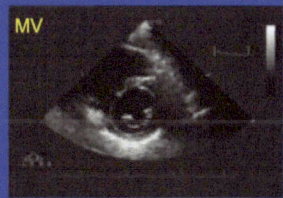
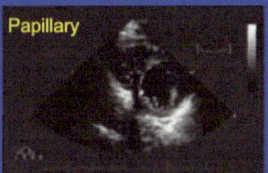 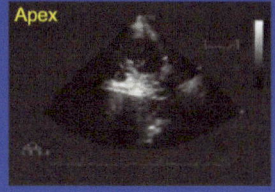

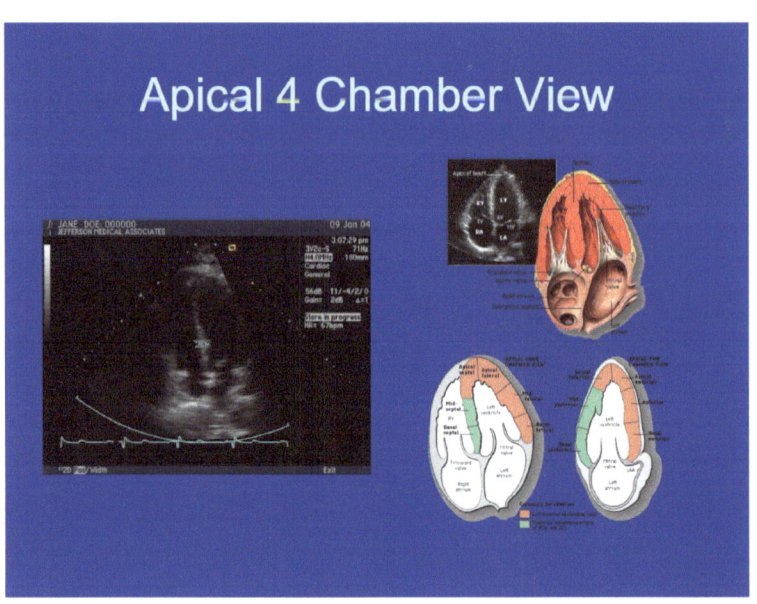

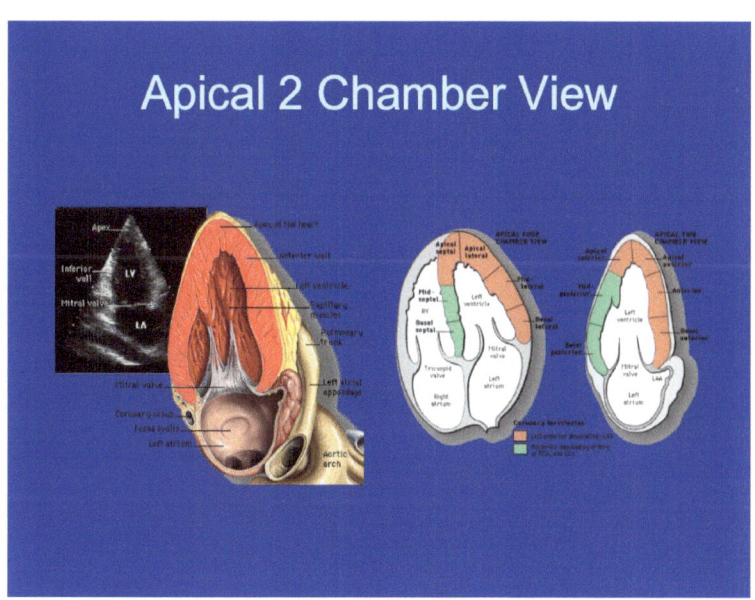

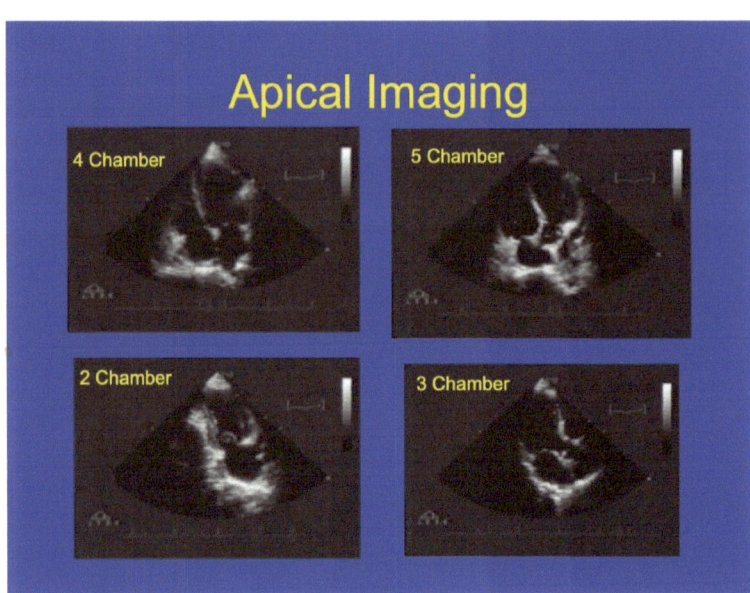

Sub-xyphoid View

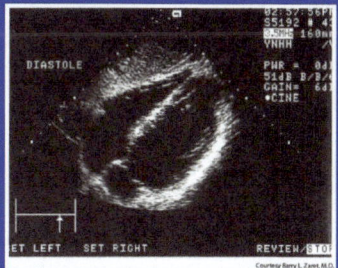
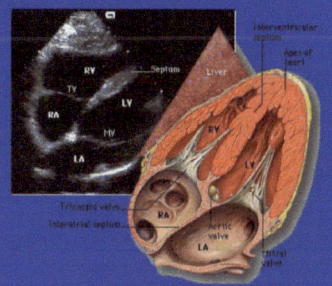

Subcostal View
IVC, Eustachian Valve & RA pressures.

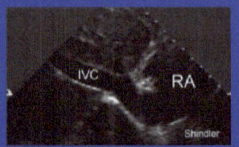

- RA pressures (inhalation or sniff)
  - IVC collapse = 5 mm Hg
  - Partial IVC collapse = 14 mm Hg
  - Non-reactive (no collapse) = 20 mm Hg

The types of Images include:
2D Echocardiography for Movement of Myocardium and Endocardium (Valves).

M-Mode for Measurements.

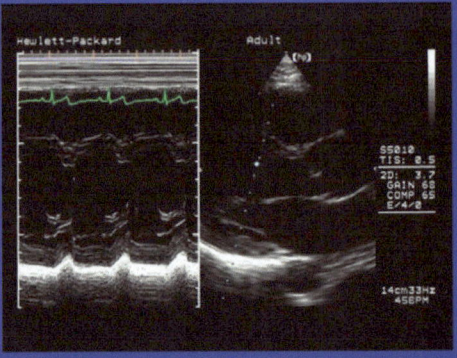

And Doppler for Velocities and Direction of Blood Movement within the Heart.

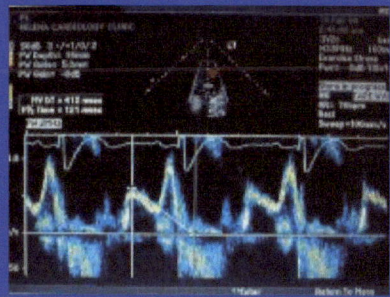 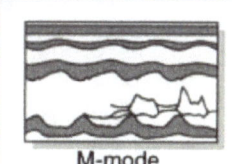

M-mode

Color Flow (The Doppler Shift).

What are you Looking for?

- Information about the atria
  - Are they larger than they should be
    - Why?
      - Stenosis or regurgitation
- Information about the ventricles
  - Are they normal or large
  - Thick or not
  - Is there a wall motion abnormality
    - Regional or diffuse

What are you Looking for?

- Is there anything wrong with the valves.
  - Hyper echoic, stenotic, regurgitant
- Are there thrombi
  - Why should there be
- Are there holes
  - ASD, VSD, perforated valves
- Pericardial effusions
  - A problem or not

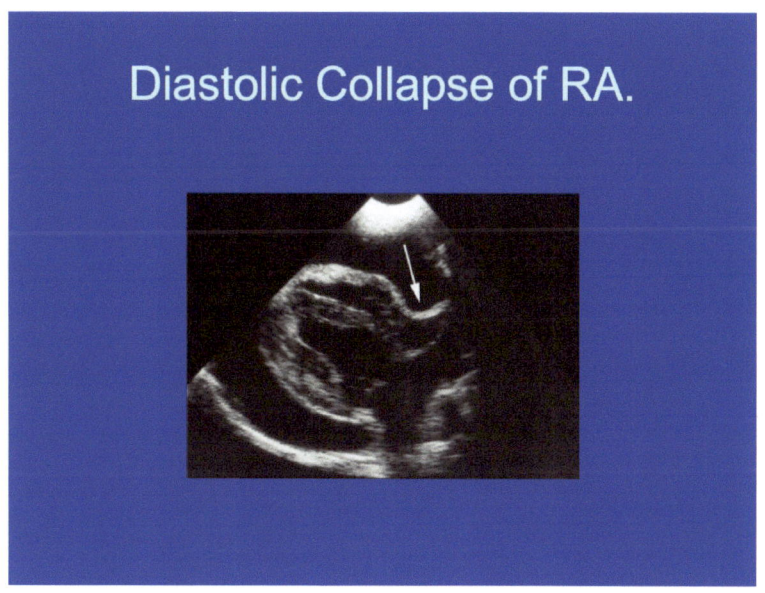

As a nurse or nursing student, having a fundamental understanding of what an echocardiogram looks like, and what we are looking for as Cardiologists, can be an invaluable tool in our communication with you about the health of the patient.

www.ingramcontent.com/pod-product-compliance
Lightning Source LLC
Chambersburg PA
CBHW041945240526
45473CB00033B/616